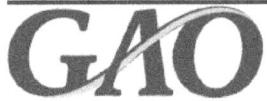

United States Government Accountability Office

Report to Congressional Committees

I0455240

November 2013

DEFENSE HEALTH CARE REFORM

Additional Implementation Details Would Increase Transparency of DOD's Plans and Enhance Accountability

DEFENSE HEALTH CARE REFORM

Additional Implementation Details Would Increase Transparency of DOD's Plans and Enhance Accountability

GAO Highlights

Highlights of GAO-14-49, a report to congressional committees

Why GAO Did This Study

Over the past decade, the cost of DOD's MHS has increased to almost $50 billion and is expected to double by 2030. Section 731 of the National Defense Authorization Act for Fiscal Year 2013 required DOD to provide three submissions detailing its plan to reform its MHS governance structure and also mandated that GAO submit an analysis of DOD's first two submissions. This report addresses the extent to which DOD's March and June 2013 submissions met the statutory requirements and reflect key management practices. GAO compared DOD's submissions for reforming its MHS governance structure with the (1) statutory requirements and (2) key management practices contained in GAO's *Business Process Reengineering Assessment Guide* and other relevant GAO work. Additionally, GAO interviewed DOD officials from the Office of the Assistant Secretary of Defense for Health Affairs, the MHS Transition Office, and the military services' Surgeons General offices.

What GAO Recommends

To provide decision makers with more complete information on the implementation of DOD's newly created DHA, GAO recommends that DOD develop and present to Congress fully developed performance measures, interim timelines, and staffing baseline assessments, and refined cost savings estimates. In written responses to this report, DOD concurred with each of GAO's recommendations.

View GAO-14-49. For more information, contact Brenda S. Farrell at 202-512-3604 or farrellb@gao.gov.

What GAO Found

GAO determined that the Department of Defense's (DOD) March and June 2013 submissions on establishing a Defense Health Agency (DHA) to reform the governance of the Military Health System (MHS) met three statutory requirements to include information on goals, performance measures, and staffing; partially met one requirement to include information on timelines; and was not required to include information on shared services because the reporting time frame was not applicable. GAO also assessed the submissions to determine the extent to which DOD incorporated key management practices from GAO's prior work on business-process reengineering. DOD's submissions provided some useful information but did not fully incorporate some key management practices as explained below.

- DOD presented 87 performance measures under its seven goals for its MHS reform. However, those measures do not fully exhibit the attributes of successful performance measures that can help agencies determine whether they are achieving their goals as well as identify areas for improvement. Examples of key attributes include clarity, measurable targets, and baseline data. None of DOD's measures included an accompanying explanation, definition, or a quantifiable target nor did they include information regarding relevant baseline assessments.

- DOD provided a list of major governance milestones and an overall schedule for activities related to establishing the DHA. However, DOD's implementation timeline did not include interim milestones for four of the seven goals of its reform. A key practice for agencies undergoing business transformations is to develop a detailed implementation plan with milestones for all actions so that progress can be closely monitored.

- In its June submission, DOD provided an estimate of authorized staff needed as of October 1, 2013, for the DHA. However, DOD does not have the information to determine how the creation of the DHA will affect the total number of MHS headquarters staff because it has not completed an updated baseline assessment of current staffing levels. Key management practices require agencies to be aware of the size, knowledge, skills, and abilities of their workforces to pursue their missions. DOD planned to submit revised estimated staffing levels in a September 30, 2013 submission to Congress.

- DOD presented business cases that included a breakdown of estimated implementation costs and aggregated cost-savings estimates for the consolidation of four shared services. However, some key details of a sound business case were missing, such as the basis for the savings. DOD's business cases aggregated the separate business lines of its shared services, which obscures the size and cost of planned efficiencies for each discrete business line, and it did not assess the risk that implementation costs could increase.

Without more clear, complete, and transparent information on DOD's plan for establishment of the DHA, it will be difficult for decision makers to gauge progress and identify areas of risk that will need to be monitored during implementation.

_____ **United States Government Accountability Office**

Contents

Abbreviations

DHA	Defense Health Agency
DOD	Department of Defense
JTF CAPMED	Joint Task Force National Capital Region Medical
MHS	Military Health System
OASD HA	Office of the Assistant Secretary of Defense for Health Affairs

GAO U.S. GOVERNMENT ACCOUNTABILITY OFFICE

441 G St. N.W.
Washington, DC 20548

November 6, 2013

Congressional Committees

On October 1, 2013, the Department of Defense (DOD) established a
new Defense Health Agency (DHA) to assume management
responsibility of numerous functions of its medical health care system.
This change comes after a long series of studies since 1949 addressing
the issue of the governance structure of DOD's Military Health System
(MHS). DOD faces increasing pressure on its budgetary resources, and in
a March 2013 memorandum directing the establishment of a DHA, the
Secretary of Defense noted that DOD needs to be responsive to current
fiscal challenges facing the nation. Over the past decade, the Defense
Health Program budget has grown substantially, from $19 billion in fiscal
year 2001 to the fiscal year 2014 budget request of $49.4 billion. Further,
the Congressional Budget Office has projected MHS costs to reach about
$92 billion by 2030. As health care consumes an increasingly large
portion of the defense budget, DOD leadership has acknowledged the
need to reduce duplication and overhead, operate its health system as
efficiently as possible, and realize savings in the MHS through the
adoption of common clinical and business processes. In recent years,
numerous sources such as the Defense Business Board in 2006,[1]
Defense Health Board in 2007,[2] and DOD-initiated internal efficiency

---

[1]The Defense Business Board stated that DOD may not be fulfilling its obligations under
public law requiring consolidation of shared services. Defense Business Board, *Military
Health System-Governance, Alignment and Configuration of Business Activities Task
Group Report*, Report to the Secretary of Defense, Report FY06-5, September 2006.

[2]The Defense Health Board noted in its 2007 report that although consolidation and
centralization are occurring at the military service level, fragmentation still exists at the
MHS enterprise level. Defense Health Board, *Task Force on the Future of Military Health
Care Final Report*, December 2007.

reviews,[3] as well as our previous reviews of DOD's medical governance,[4] have identified areas for reform of DOD's health care system. As a result, DOD established the DHA and chartered an implementation planning team consisting of officials from throughout the MHS to provide continuing oversight, management direction, and support of this reform.

Following DOD's 2012 decision to implement this reform to the governance of the MHS, the National Defense Authorization Act for Fiscal Year 2013 required that DOD create a detailed implementation plan for carrying out its health care system reform, and provide it to the congressional defense committees in three separate submissions in fiscal year 2013. In a submission due no later than March 31, 2013, Congress required DOD to provide goals it is to achieve while carrying out the reform along with a detailed schedule to carry out the reform, including a schedule for meeting its goals. In a second submission, due no later than June 30, 2013, Congress required DOD to provide metrics to evaluate the achievement of each goal, the required personnel levels, and specific information on the shared services[5] that DOD planned to implement during fiscal year 2013. In the third submission, due no later than September 30, 2013, Congress required DOD to provide details concerning the shared services it planned to implement during fiscal year 2014. DOD provided its first submission to the congressional defense committees on March 15, 2013, and its second submission on June 27, 2013.

---

[3]The Secretary of Defense directed a series of initiatives to move the defense enterprise toward a more efficient, effective, and cost-conscious way of doing business, in part, by reducing excess and duplication. See, for example, Secretary of Defense Memorandum, *Department of Defense (DOD) Efficiency Initiatives*, Memorandum (Aug. 16, 2010) and Secretary of Defense Memorandum, *Track Four Efficiency Initiatives Decisions*, Memorandum (Mar. 14, 2011).

[4]GAO, *Defense Health Care: DOD Needs to Address the Expected Benefits, Costs, and Risks for Its Newly Approved Medical Command Structure*, GAO-08-122 (Washington, D.C.: Oct. 12, 2007); *Defense Health Care: Applying Key Management Practices Should Help Achieve Efficiencies within the Military Health System*, GAO-12-224 *(Washington, D.C.: Apr. 12, 2012); Defense Health Care: Additional Analysis of Costs and Benefits of Potential Governance Structures Is Needed*, GAO-12-911 (Washington, D.C.: Sept. 26, 2012).

[5]According to DOD, a shared services concept is a combination of common services performed across the medical community. DOD identified 10 shared services it plans to implement: medical logistics, facility planning, health information technology, health plan management, pharmacy, medical education and training, medical research and development, public health, acquisition, and budget and resource management.

The National Defense Authorization Act for Fiscal Year 2013 further required that GAO submit to the congressional defense committees a review of the contents of the first two submissions of DOD's plan to assess whether DOD met the statutory requirements. In May 2013, we provided a briefing to the committees on information that included the extent to which DOD's March 2013 first submission on its plan for MHS governance reform contained the statutorily required elements of goals and a schedule for achievement of those goals. We also included our preliminary observations on how well DOD's goals linked to the proposed responsibilities of its new DHA and how the schedule could be improved by incorporating features that we have found to be useful in effective planning for achieving performance and cost-savings goals. As a result of that briefing to the House Armed Services Committee personnel, the House Report accompanying a bill for the National Defense Authorization Act for Fiscal Year 2014 included language that directed the Secretary of Defense to provide the House Armed Services Committee with additional information to address the shortcomings that we had identified. DOD provided additional information to respond to the shortcomings we had identified regarding DOD's first submission in its June 2013 second submission and a supplemental report to the committee on August 16, 2013. For this report, we are consolidating the results of our review of both DOD's March and June 2013 submissions to Congress. Accordingly, our objective for this report was to determine to what extent DOD's March and June 2013 medical governance submissions address statutory requirements and reflect key management practices.

To determine the extent to which DOD's March and June 2013 submissions of its plan to reform its MHS governance address the statutory requirements, we obtained and reviewed both of DOD's submissions to the congressional defense committees and the elements required by the National Defense Authorization Act for Fiscal Year 2013. We compared the two to determine the submissions' compliance with the statutory requirements. We rated compliance for each requirement as "addressed," "partially addressed," or "not addressed." We considered the requirement to be "addressed" in the submission when DOD explicitly addressed all parts set forth in the requirement. We considered the requirement "partially addressed" in the submission when DOD addressed at least one or more, but not all, parts of the requirement. We considered the requirement "not addressed" by DOD when the submission did not explicitly address any part of the requirement. Further, to determine the extent to which these medical governance submissions reflected key management practices as identified in GAO's *Business Process Reengineering Assessment Guide* and other leading practices we have identified in our prior work,[6] we focused our review specifically on the information contained in the March and June 2013 medical governance submissions DOD submitted to Congress. Using our prior work that identified key management practices and key characteristics of effective planning for achieving performance and cost-savings goals, we determined whether DOD's March and June 2013 submissions included information consistent with those practices or characteristics. Additionally, we analyzed DOD's August 16, 2013, supplemental report[7] to determine if the information it provided was consistent with our identified key management practices. Further, we conducted interviews with officials, including those from the Office of the Assistant Secretary of Defense for Health Affairs (OASD HA), the MHS Governance Transition Office, the Offices of the Surgeons General for the Army, the Navy, and the Air Force, and the TRICARE Management Activity to clarify how DOD's submissions were developed and to understand the structure that DOD has established to manage its transition to a DHA.

We conducted this performance audit from March 2013 to November 2013 in accordance with generally accepted government auditing standards. Those standards require that we plan and perform the audit to obtain sufficient, appropriate evidence to provide a reasonable basis for our findings and conclusions based on our audit objectives. We believe that the evidence obtained provides a reasonable basis for our findings and conclusions based on our audit objectives.

Background

The MHS is a complex organization that provides health services to almost 10 million beneficiaries across a range of care venues, including the battlefield, traditional hospitals and clinics at stationary locations, and authorized civilian providers. As we reported in 2005, DOD's health care system is an example of a key challenge facing the U.S. government in

---

[6]GAO, *Business Process Reengineering Assessment Guide*, GAO/AIMD-10.1.15 (May 1997); *Streamlining Government: Questions to Consider When Evaluating Proposals to Consolidate Physical Infrastructure and Management Functions*, GAO-12-542 (Washington, D.C.: May 23, 2012); GAO-12-224.

[7]Subsequent to DOD's March submission, the House Report accompanying the proposed National Defense Authorization Act for Fiscal Year 2014 directed the Secretary of Defense to provide the House Armed Services Committee with additional information about the DHA's milestones and goals. In response, DOD submitted a supplemental report on August 16, 2013.

the 21st century as well as an area in which DOD can achieve economies of scale and improve delivery by combining, realigning, or otherwise changing selected support functions.[8] Additionally, in 2011, we reported that the responsibilities and authorities for DOD's military health system were distributed among several organizations within DOD with no central command authority or single entity accountable for minimizing costs and achieving efficiencies.[9] Under the MHS command structure that existed prior to October 1, 2013, the OASD HA, the Army, the Navy, and the Air Force each had its own headquarters and associated support functions, such as information technology, human capital management, financial activities, and contracting. Additionally, the three services' Surgeons General were responsible for overseeing their deployable medical forces and operating their health care systems.[10] OASD HA manages the Defense Health Program budget, but this office does not directly supervise the services' medical personnel. See figure 1 for the organizational structure prior to October 1, 2013.[11]

[8]GAO, *21st Century Challenges: Reexamining the Base of the Federal Government,* GAO-05-325SP (Washington, D.C.: February 2005).

[9]GAO, *Opportunities to Reduce Potential Duplication in Government Programs, Save Tax Dollars, and Enhance Revenue,* GAO-11-318SP (Washington, D.C.: Mar. 1, 2011).

[10]With the creation of the DHA, the services' Surgeons General will continue to be responsble for overseeing medical forces and operating health care systems including Military Treatment Facilities.

[11]Under the new governance structure, the Assistant Secretary of Defense for Health Affairs will maintain these same responsibilities.

Figure 1: Organizational Structure of the Military Health System Prior to October 1, 2013

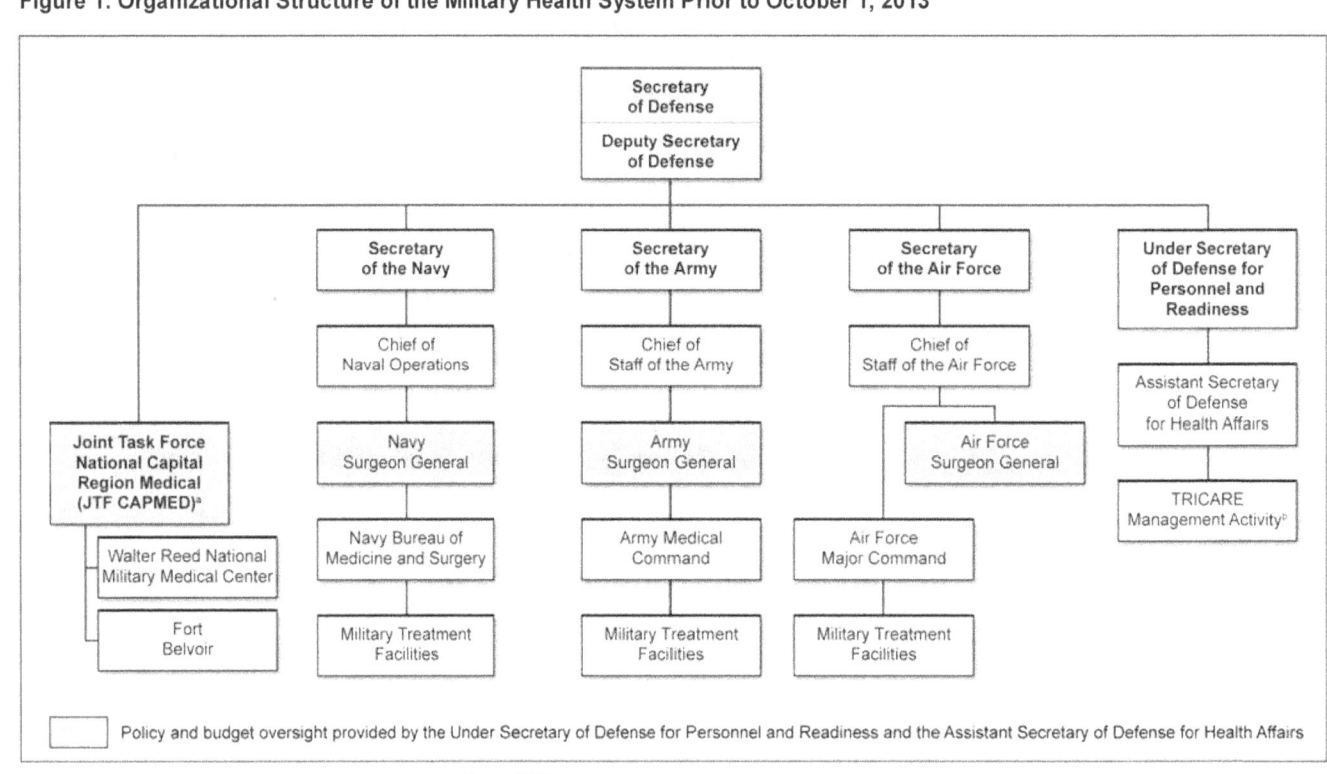

Source: DOD.

[a]The Joint Task Force National Capital Region Medical (JTF CAPMED) was an additional medical organizational structure and reporting chain that was established in 2007 to manage the Military Treatment Facilities within the National Capital Region and the execution of related 2005 Base Realignment and Closure actions in that area. The JTF CAPMED and its Commander reported to the Secretary of Defense through the Deputy Secretary of Defense. The two inpatient medical facilities in the area, Walter Reed National Military Medical Center and Fort Belvoir Community Hospital, were directed by the Deputy Secretary of Defense in January 2009 to become joint commands.

[b]DOD provides civilian health care to millions of eligible beneficiaries through its TRICARE program, which was managed by the TRICARE Management Activity prior to October 1, 2013.

Over the years, many efforts to control the increase in health care costs led to a long series of studies to address the governance structure of the MHS and to recommend major organizational realignments. Most recently, in March 2011, the Deputy Secretary of Defense established an internal task force to conduct a review of the governance of the MHS. The task force identified (1) cost containment, (2) greater integration, and (3) increased unity of effort as priority objectives for the MHS. The task force's September 2011 report noted the need for clear decision authority and accountability. Following numerous internal discussions, DOD submitted a report to Congress in March 2012 outlining various options for reforming the MHS governance, including creating a DHA. Additionally, at that time, the Deputy Secretary of Defense directed DOD leadership to develop an implementation plan that would center on the establishment of a DHA. As a result of that direction, the department began implementation planning for this change, including organizational changes.

MHS Governance Transition Organization Chartered to Direct Reform

To help ensure that the department maintained momentum on this reform, the Deputy Secretary of Defense directed the formation of a team to develop an implementation plan for the governance changes. As a result, the Assistant Secretary of Defense for Health Affairs established a chartered MHS Governance Transition Organization to provide oversight, management, and support for the implementation of MHS governance reforms in March 2013.[12] This transition organization consists of individuals, an action group, an advisory council, along with a review board, each with specific roles and responsibilities. This organization is chartered to exist until October 2015, when the DHA is expected to reach full operating capability. The formation of this MHS Governance Transition Organization addresses a concern that we expressed to DOD in a previous report[13] about how DOD did not form an overarching team to manage the implementation of a 2006 attempt to institute changes to its medical governance structure. See figure 2 for a diagram of the MHS Governance Transition Organization.

[12]The MHS Governance Transition Organization Charter was signed on March 25, 2013.

[13]GAO-12-224.

Figure 2: Military Health System Governance Transition Organizational Structure

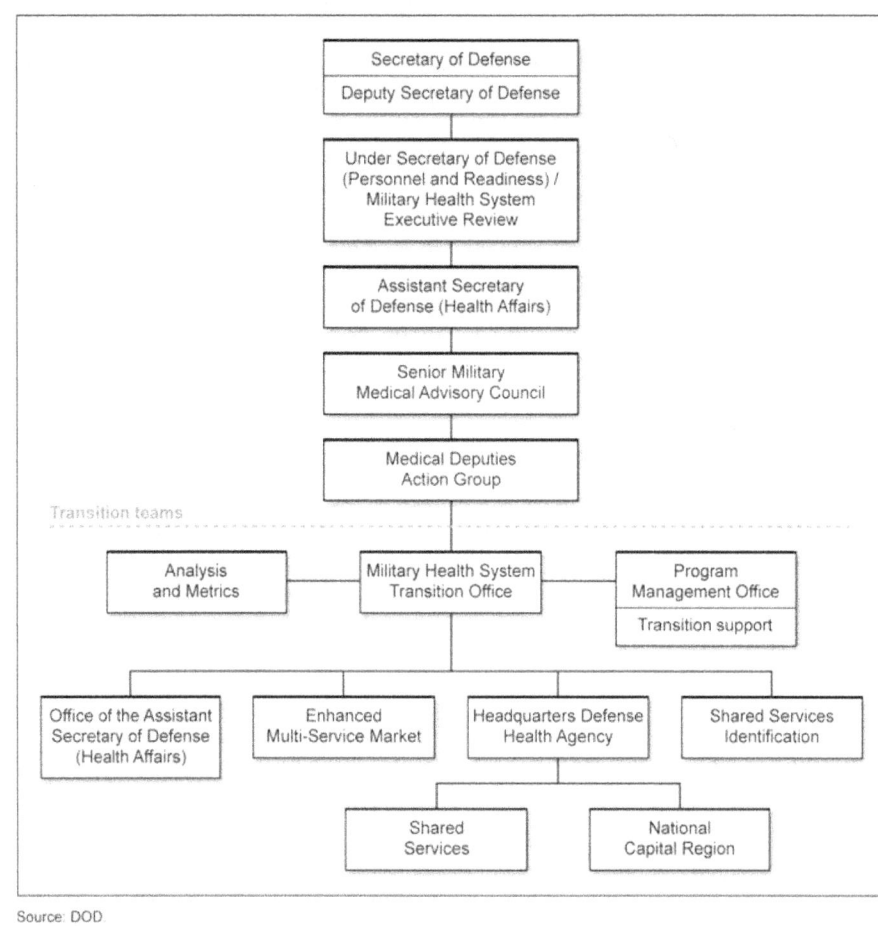

Source: DOD

The roles and responsibilities of the primary leaders within the MHS for overseeing the governance reform are as follows:

- The Deputy Secretary of Defense serves as the final decision maker on all changes to MHS governance.

- The Under Secretary of Defense for Personnel and Readiness will approve the implementation plans.

- The Military Health System Executive Review, which is chaired by the Under Secretary of Defense for Personnel and Readiness and has other members such as the Vice Chiefs of Staff for the three services as well as the Director of the Joint Staff, will provide a forum for

GAO-14-49 DOD's 2013 Medical Governance Plans

dispute resolution and oversight of MHS governance transition and implementation activities.

- The Assistant Secretary of Defense for Health Affairs is accountable for the overall management and direction of the MHS Governance Transition Organization.

- The Senior Military Medical Advisory Council, which is chaired by the Assistant Secretary of Defense for Health Affairs and includes the service Surgeons General and others, will review, recommend, and advise the Assistant Secretary of Defense for Health Affairs on service-specific implementation issues.

- The Medical Deputies Action Group, which consists of the service Deputy Surgeons General, the Joint Staff Surgeon, and a DHA representative, and is chaired by the Principal Deputy Assistant Secretary of Defense for Health Affairs, provides oversight of the detailed activities of the transition office and its subordinate transition teams.

- The MHS Governance Transition Office provides oversight of day-to-day implementation activities, to include such actions as (1) integrating all transition teams' activities; (2) compiling all implementation costs, cost savings, and cost avoidance that result from transition activities, and (3) updating higher management at least weekly on progress and issues, and developing reports, presentations, and other necessary documents.

DHA Organizational Structure Establishes Centralized Accountability for Consolidated Shared Services

The MHS Governance Transition Organization with its component parts is working to implement the governance reforms laid out by the Deputy Secretary of Defense to establish the DHA that will support the execution of policy, manage the military's health plan, manage medical operations within the National Capital Region,[14] and provide shared services. In doing so, the DHA will support the services in execution of their medical missions. See figure 3 below for the organizational chart of the proposed DHA.

---

[14] The National Capital Region is the geographic area that includes Washington, D.C., and other specific surrounding cities and counties in both Maryland and Virginia.

Figure 3: Proposed Defense Health Agency Organizational Chart

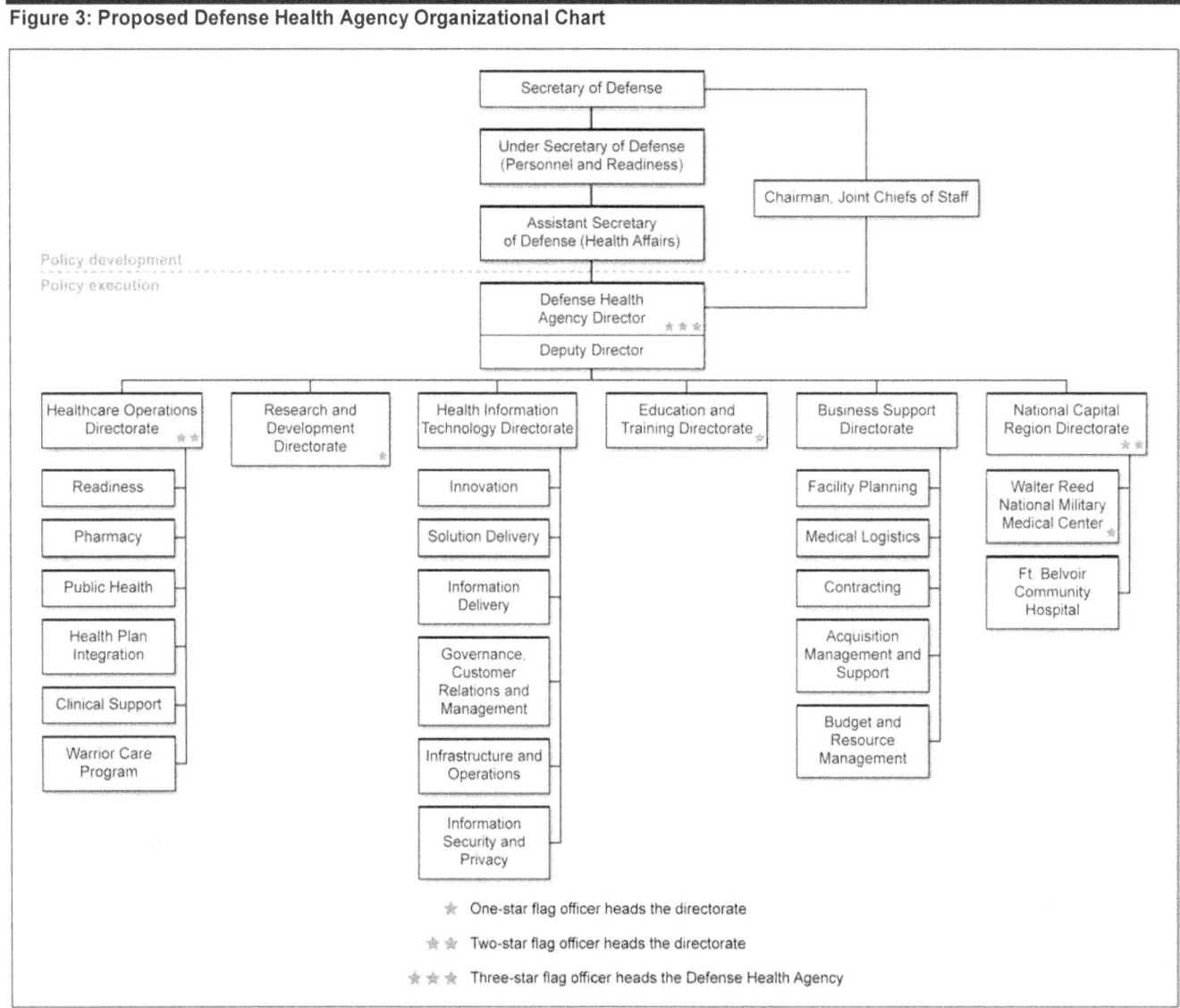

Source: DOD

Officials discussed the proposed DHA organization with us and provided general descriptions of the subordinate directorates shown in figure 3. According to these officials,

- the proposed Healthcare Operations Directorate would manage MHS operations in such areas as pharmacy, public health issues, the warrior care program, clinical support, readiness, and the health plan for beneficiaries;

- the proposed Research and Development Directorate would manage MHS operations in the area of medical research and development issues;

- the proposed Health Information Technology Directorate would manage MHS operations in such areas as information security and privacy, information delivery, infrastructure and operations, and innovation;

- the proposed Education and Training Directorate would manage MHS operations in the area of medical education and training for all MHS personnel;

- the proposed Business Support Directorate would manage MHS operations in such areas as facility planning, medical logistics, budget and resources management, acquisition management, and contracting; and

- the proposed National Capital Region Directorate would exercise authority, direction, and control over the inpatient facilities and subordinate clinics to deliver healthcare to eligible beneficiaries— military personnel and their dependents, eligible National Guard and Reserve personnel and their dependents, and retirees and their dependents and survivors—in the National Capital Region.

According to DOD's March and June 2013 medical governance submissions to Congress, its plan to reform the MHS governance structure is intended to further integrate its health care delivery system and to enhance the way resources and care are coordinated and redistributed across a variety of delivery sites to best address population needs. In 2003 the Under Secretary of Defense for Personnel and Readiness designated responsibilities and authorities for Multi-Service Markets,[15] which included common appointment processes, referral management, and capacity and workload planning. DOD's June 2013 submission states that the initial attempts to implement this concept

---

[15]Multi-Service Markets are areas in which more than one DOD component provides military health care services.

demonstrated some success. Further, DOD's first submission states that substantial improvements in clinical and business processes will occur, and major reductions in cost through standardized processes and recapture of private-sector care are most achievable at this multiservice market level. As such, DOD has designated six areas throughout the country as enhanced Multi-Service Markets[16] that will implement 5-year performance plans to produce improvements in clinical and business practices and cost, infrastructure, and personnel reductions. The details of how these improvements will be achieved and their yearly cost and performance targets are to be specified in performance plans that are to be submitted to the Assistant Secretary of Defense (Health Affairs) through both the Medical Deputies Action Group and the Senior Military Medical Advisory Council as part of the MHS governance reform. Additionally, because the enhanced Multi-Service Markets managers will be accountable for performance of military treatment facilities operated by more than one military service, DOD has reported that it has established a new governance structure with representation from the three services, and the DHA has been implemented to provide oversight for the planning, implementation, and execution of business performance plans.

A final component of the new DHA is the establishment of the National Capital Region Directorate. According to DOD, this arrangement keeps the joint organizational structure of the two inpatient hospitals within the National Capital Region—Walter Reed National Military Medical Center at Bethesda and Fort Belvoir Community Hospital—as well as allowing a reduction to the number of intermediate-level headquarters' overhead positions.

---

[16]The six multiservice markets identified are Tidewater, Virginia; Colorado Springs, Colorado; San Antonio, Texas; Puget Sound, Washington; Hawaii; and the National Capital Region.

DOD's Submissions for Its MHS Reform Largely Met Statutory Requirements but Did Not Fully Incorporate Some Key Management Practices

The National Defense Authorization Act for Fiscal Year 2013 required that DOD's first two submissions on health care governance reform to Congress include (1) goals to achieve while carrying out the reform, (2) performance measures to evaluate the achievement of each goal, (3) the required personnel levels, (4) a detailed schedule for carrying out reform goals including a schedule for meeting the goals, and (5) detailed information in a business-case analysis for each shared service to be implemented during fiscal year 2013. In its March and June 2013 submissions of its plan for the MHS governance reform, DOD addressed the first three statutory requirements, partially addressed the fourth, and was not required to address the last item. Specifically, in its submissions, DOD presented (1) one overall and seven subordinate goals of its reform, (2) performance measures it plans to use to evaluate the achievement of each of the goals, and (3) an estimate of the personnel levels required for the DHA. However, DOD partially addressed its statutory requirement to provide information about its schedule for carrying out the reform because it presented milestones for only four of the seven subordinate goals. Lastly, the statute required DOD to present detailed information in a business-case analysis for each shared service that was implemented during fiscal year 2013. However, DOD did not plan to implement any shared services in fiscal year 2013, and thus it was not required by statute to provide business case analyses for any shared services. Nonetheless, DOD included a discussion of the first four shared services it plans to implement in fiscal year 2014, which were medical logistics, facilities planning, health information technology, and the health care plan. DOD was required to submit a third submission in September 2013 that would address its business-case analyses for shared services to be implemented in fiscal year 2014.

In addition to determining whether DOD's submissions addressed the statutory requirements, we determined the extent to which DOD incorporated key management practices derived from GAO's past work into its March and June 2013 submissions. DOD's submissions of its plan for MHS governance reform provided some useful information but did not fully incorporate some key management practices that we have found promote effective planning, implementation, and oversight in managing successful business-process reengineering. In discussing DOD's required submissions with officials, they said that they followed the guidance in our *Business Process Reengineering Assessment Guide* as they moved forward. This guide covers a wide range of activities, such as identifying mission and goals, establishing performance measures to gauge progress, developing a sound business case for implementing the new process, and identifying appropriate staffing levels.[17] DOD's submissions do reflect some of these practices, including information on how DOD believes the goals for the reform would result in improvements and savings within the MHS and high-level business-case analyses for its efficiency efforts. However, DOD's submissions did not fully incorporate these key management practices because they did not include clear, quantifiable, objective performance measures and a baseline assessment of current performance; interim timelines for meeting four of the seven goals; complete implementation costs for its business-case analyses for shared services; and estimated personnel levels for full operating capability. The inclusion of such information would help more-fully explain how DOD intends to implement and oversee this significant transition.

Some of DOD's Goals Presented in Its March 2013 Submission Were Not Clearly Linked to the Responsibilities of the DHA but Were Later Clarified

DOD's March 2013 submission for MHS governance reform was required to contain goals to achieve while carrying out the reform—including goals with respect to improving clinical and business practices and reductions in costs, infrastructure, and personnel. In the March submission, DOD addressed this requirement by presenting the goals of the reform in the form of one overall strategic goal and seven subordinate goals. DOD's overarching strategic goal for its MHS is to achieve greater system integration. Its seven subordinate goals are as follows:

(1) promote more-effective and efficient health care operations through enhanced enterprise-wide shared services;

(2) deliver more-comprehensive primary care and integrated health services using advanced patient-centered medical homes;

(3) coordinate care over time and across treatment settings to improve outcomes in the management of chronic illness, particularly for patients with complex medical and social problems;

(4) match personnel, infrastructure, and funding to current missions, future missions, and population demand;

(5) establish more interservice standards and metrics, and standardize processes to promote learning and continuous improvement;

---

[17]GAO/AIMD-10.1.15.

(6) create enhanced value in military medical markets using an integrated approach specified in 5-year business performance plans; and,

(7) align incentives with health and readiness outcomes to reward value creation.

Although DOD met the statutory requirements to submit goals, its initial submission did not clearly show the linkage between the goals and the mission of the transformation. GAO's *Business Process Re-Engineering Assessment Guide* states that agencies should develop goals that are clearly linked to the agency's mission and what needs to be accomplished to help challenge and motivate an agency to modify its performance.[18] According to DOD's submissions, the strategic vision of the MHS transformation is "to deliver a coordinated continuum of preventive and curative services to eligible beneficiaries and be accountable for health outcomes and cost while supporting the services' warfighter requirements." DOD has stated that it selected the DHA to be the organizational structure that will allow the department to achieve this mission by accelerating the implementation of shared services with common clinical and business practices.

We found that three of DOD's subordinate goals—(1) promote more-effective and efficient health care operations through enhanced enterprise-wide shared services; (2) establish more interservice standards/metrics, and standardize processes to promote learning and continuous improvement; and (3) create enhanced value in military medical markets using an integrated approach specified in 5-year business performance plans—were clearly linked to the establishment of the DHA in that it was clear how the new agency would be responsible for implementing or supporting these goals. However, we found that the remaining four subordinate goals—(1) deliver more-comprehensive primary care and integrated health services using advanced patient-centered medical homes; (2) coordinate care over time and across treatment settings to improve outcomes in the management of chronic illness, particularly for patients with complex medical and social problems; (3) match personnel, infrastructure, and funding to current missions, future missions, and population demand; and, (4) align incentives with health and readiness outcomes to reward value creation—did not clearly link to the DHA's proposed responsibilities, because either the

---

[18]GAO/AIMD-10.1.15.

responsibilities stemming from the four subordinate goals already belong to the services or the goal is not clearly defined. Moreover, in some cases, the function could be achieved regardless of the existence of the DHA. For example, one of the goals is to deliver more-comprehensive primary care and integrated health services using advanced patient-centered medical homes. However, the services are responsible for delivering all primary care, and as such, DOD officials told us that each service began implementing its own patient-centered medical homes model approximately 3 years prior to the establishment of the DHA as a means to address concerns in growing dissatisfaction with patient care. Another goal of the reform is to coordinate care over time and across treatment settings to improve outcomes in the management of chronic illness, particularly for patients with complex medical and social problems. However, this function was already being performed prior to the establishment of the DHA, as the services are currently responsible for coordinating care across treatment settings.

Subsequent to DOD's submission of its goals in its March 2013 submission and our May 2013 congressional briefing on our preliminary observations of this submission, the House Report accompanying the proposed National Defense Authorization Act for Fiscal Year 2014 directed the Secretary of Defense to provide the House Armed Services Committee with more information concerning how DOD developed its goals and to clarify the linkage of the goals to the responsibilities of the newly formed DHA. DOD responded to this direction by providing additional details in its June 2013 submission that were absent from its March 2013 submission. Specifically, DOD explained who derived and approved the goals, what responsibilities the new DHA would have in achieving its goals, and how clinical and business practices would be improved with the creation of the DHA, as well as what cost, infrastructure, and personnel reductions could be expected from this reform. In the June submission, DOD stated the seven goals were derived and endorsed by the MHS leadership, including the Surgeons General of the services. In addition, DOD provided an explanation as to how each goal related to the DHA. For instance, DOD explained that implementation of the patient-centered medical home model on a service-specific basis had resulted in significant clinical and business process variation among the services, along with use of different metrics. According to DOD's June 2013 submission, the DHA will standardize the patient-centered medical home model through, among other means, the DHA Health Care Operations Directorate, which will monitor enterprise performance with measures applied consistently across the services, such as standardized business processes for appointments and referral management. In addition, in its June 2013 submission, DOD provided an explanation of the clinical and business-practice improvements and cost, infrastructure, and personnel reductions to be realized for each goal. For instance, a DOD study found a significant positive effect on various cost and utilization metrics at three patient-centered medical home implementation sites, including lower utilization rates of inpatient services, emergency room, and urgent care services, with decreases in per member per month costs. In its June 2013 submission, DOD explained that on the basis of this study, it anticipates that using the DHA to monitor, evaluate, and promulgate patient-centered medical home successes should result in costs reductions across the Military Health System.

DOD Addressed Statutory Requirement to Provide Performance Measures; However, the Measures Do Not Fully Meet Best Practices

DOD's June 2013 submission was required to include performance measures to evaluate the achievement of each reform goal with respect to the purpose, objective, and improvements made by each goal. We found that DOD addressed this requirement because it listed in its June 2013 submission 87 different performance measures aligned under the seven subordinate goals.[19] However, in analyzing the measures DOD included in the submission, we found those measures do not exhibit important attributes of successful performance measures that we established in our prior work. We have previously reported[20] that federal agencies engaging in large projects, including consolidating management functions, can use performance measures to determine how well they are achieving their goals and identify areas for improvement, if needed. Additionally, we have found that by tracking and developing a performance baseline for all measures, agencies can better evaluate progress made and whether or not goals are being achieved. By using performance measures, ongoing monitoring, and reporting on activities in a transparent manner, key decision makers can obtain feedback for improving both policy and operational effectiveness. Identifying and reporting deviations from the baseline as a program proceeds provides valuable information for oversight by identifying areas of program risk and their causes to decision makers. Through our prior work on performance

---

[19]Some performance measures were used to assess multiple objectives.

[20]GAO-12-542.

measurement, we have identified several important attributes of performance measures (see table 1).[21]

Table 1: Attributes of Performance Measures

Attribute	Definition
Balance	A suite of measures ensures that an organization's various priorities are covered.
Clarity	Measure is clearly stated, and the name and definition are consistent with the methodology used to calculate it.
Core program activities	Measures cover the activities that an entity is expected to perform to support the intent of the program.
Government-wide priorities	Each measure covers a priority such as quality, timeliness, and cost of service.
Limited overlap	Measures provide new information beyond that provided by other measures.
Linkage	Measure is aligned with division and agency-wide goals and mission and is clearly communicated throughout the organization.
Measurable target	Measure has a numerical goal.
Objectivity	Measure is reasonably free from significant bias or manipulation.
Reliability	Measure produces the same result under similar conditions.
Baseline and Trend Data	Measure has a baseline and trend data associated with it to identify, monitor, and report changes in performance and to help ensure that performance is viewed in context.

Source: GAO.

In its June 2013 submission, DOD listed 87 performance measures to assess its seven goals, and provided only the measures' names with no accompanying explanation, definition, or a quantifiable, numerical target for performance. For example, DOD listed "HEDIS preventive measures" as a performance measure without an accompanying explanation or definition. Another measure DOD listed was "TRICARE Service Centers," which does not indicate specifically what aspect of the service centers is to be observed and measured. Further, decision makers using the submission will be unable to determine to what extent there is overlap among the measures because DOD did not provide an explanation of what each measure will evaluate, which could be used to determine

[21]GAO, *Tax Administration: IRS Needs to Further Refine Its Tax Filing Season Performance Measures,* GAO-03-143 (Washington, D.C.: Nov. 22, 2002); *GPRA Performance Reports,* GAO/GGD-96-66R, (Washington, D.C.: Feb. 14, 1996); *Missile Defense: Opportunity to Refocus on Strengthening Acquisition Management,* GAO-13-432 (Washington, D.C.: Apr. 26, 2013); *Performance Measurement and Evaluation: Definitions and Relationships,* GAO-11-646SP (Washington, D.C.: May 2011); and *Agency Performance Plans: Examples of Practices That Can Improve Usefulness to Decisionmakers,* GAO/GGD/AIMD-99-69 (Washington, D.C.: Feb. 26, 1999).

whether the measures provide new information beyond that provided by other measures. For example, two of the measures listed under its second goal are "satisfaction with provider communications" and "satisfaction with health care." As presented in the submission, it is not possible to determine whether there is any overlap between these measures, because the aspects of satisfaction are not clarified by any accompanying explanation. In addition, decision makers will not be able to determine the objectivity of DOD's measures because there is no information accompanying the measures that indicates specifically what is to be observed, in which population or conditions, and in what time frame. Such information would allow them to determine whether the measures are reasonably free from significant bias or manipulation. For example, one of the measures is "savings achieved versus savings projected." This measure does not indicate specifically how savings will be measured, nor does it indicate what time frame will be used to compare what savings were projected versus what was actually saved. As we have previously reported, performance measurement is the ongoing monitoring and reporting of program accomplishments, particularly progress toward preestablished goals.[22] It, additionally, involves identifying performance goals and measures, including establishing performance baselines by tracking performance over time, identifying targets for improving performance, and measuring progress against those targets.[23] In its June 2013 submission, DOD did not include numerical targets for performance or a performance baseline for its measures. DOD only listed the names of the performance measures with no accompanying information about the state of current performance or goals for performance improvement.

Senior DOD officials responded that the statute did not call for such detailed information, but instead just required the inclusion of performance metrics to evaluate the achievement of each goal. However, without such information, as well as identifying numerical targets and baseline assessments of current performance, decision makers will lack

---

[22]GAO-11-646SP.

[23]GAO, *Aviation Weather: Agencies Need to Improve Performance Measurement and Fully Address Key Challenges*, GAO-10-843, (Washington, D.C.; Sept. 9, 2010). Department of the Navy, Office of the Chief Information Officer, *Guide for Developing and Using Information Technology (IT) Performance Measurements* (Washington, D.C.: October 2001); and General Services Administration, Office of Governmentwide Policy, *Performance-Based Management: Eight Steps To Develop and Use Information Technology Performance Measures Effectively* (Washington, D.C.: 1996).

transparency over DOD's efforts to achieve change from the very start. DOD officials also explained that the proposed measures in the submission represent a mix of existing measures and measures yet to be developed or enhanced. However, they did not clearly indicate in the submission which metrics currently exist and which will need to be developed. Without transparent explanations of (1) why and how the selected performance measures are linked to specific goals, (2) the numerical targets for performance, and (3) a baseline of current performance for each measure, DOD officials and other decision makers, including members of Congress, will find it difficult to determine whether DOD's medical governance reform efforts are on track to achieve desired results or need corrective actions.

DOD's Schedule for Reform Lists Steps to Reach Initial Operating Milestone but Does Not Address Subsequent Milestones or Include Steps to Achieve All Seven Reform Goals

DOD's March 2013 submission was required to include a detailed schedule for carrying out the reform of the governance of the MHS, including a schedule for meeting the goals of the reform. In that submission, DOD provided a schedule of activities leading up to its first major milestone—initial operating capability of October 1, 2013—to establish the (1) DHA, (2) enhanced Multi-Service Markets, and (3) National Capital Region Directorate. We found that DOD partially addressed its statutory requirement to provide information about its schedule for carrying out the reform because the submission included a schedule of activities; however, it did not provide information related to activities beyond its first major milestone and it did not present milestones for achieving each of the supporting seven goals of the reform.

Moreover, the schedule presented in DOD's submission did not include some key features of effective schedules identified in our prior work, such as interim milestones or related timelines for all of the activities supporting the reform. We have found in previous work that interim milestones can be used to show progress towards implementing efforts or to make adjustments when necessary.[24] Specifically, we have reported that developing and using specific milestones and timelines to guide and gauge progress toward achieving an agency's desired results informs management of the rate of progress toward achieving goals or whether adjustments need to be made in order to maintain progress within given

---

[24]GAO/GGD/AIMD-99-69 and GAO, *Executive Guide: Effectively Implementing the Government Performance and Results Act*, GAO/GGD-96-118 (Washington, D.C.: June 1996).

time frames. Further, according to GAO's *Business Process Re-Engineering Assessment Guide*, agencies undergoing business transformations should develop a detailed implementation plan that lays out what needs to be done to achieve implementation of the new process by identifying milestones and specifying timetables for all actions so that progress can be closely monitored. However, DOD's March 2013 submission did not include these important interim milestones that help measure progress being made to reach goals. For example, while DOD's submission included a series of actions to be completed to establish the DHA by October 1, 2013—the initial operating capacity date—it provided only one milestone respectively for the establishment of the enhanced Multi-Service Markets and the National Capital Region Directorate by that date, but no interim actions or milestones that could help monitor the progress of those efforts. In addition, the submissions did not contain any interim actions or milestones between October 1, 2013, and October 1, 2015—the planned final operating capacity date. Furthermore, the schedule provided in the submission does not clearly establish how each of the supporting seven goals of the reform will be met. While a senior DOD official explained to us how the schedule's activities relate to each goal, this is not laid out in the submission itself. For instance, one of the goals is to deliver more-comprehensive primary care and integrated health services using advanced patient-centered medical homes. However, it is unclear from the submission how the timeline as presented relates to this goal because none of the dates in the schedule refer to patient-centered medical homes.

Subsequent to DOD's submission of the schedule in its March 2013 submission, the House Report accompanying the proposed National Defense Authorization Act for Fiscal Year 2014 directed the Secretary of Defense to provide the House Armed Services Committee with a detailed schedule for managing the reform effort. In response, DOD submitted a supplemental report on August 16, 2013, that included estimated interim milestones for the achievement of three of the reform goals that it had not initially provided in either of its earlier submissions. However, with respect to the four goals that milestones were provided for in the March 2013 submission, DOD only provided milestones leading up to initial operating capability. In the August supplemental report, DOD has not identified interim milestones necessary from initial operating capability to achieve full operating capability. Unless DOD develops interim milestones for its reform timelines, it may not be able to adequately monitor its progress toward achieving its goals by 2015.

DOD's Cost-Savings Estimates Presented for Shared Services Generally Reflect Key Characteristics of Business-Case Analyses, but Do Not Provide Critical Details Concerning Cost Savings

DOD's June 2013 submission was required to include detailed information in a business-case analysis for each shared service that was to be implemented during fiscal year 2013. However, DOD did not implement any shared services in fiscal year 2013, and thus it was not required by statute to provide business-case analyses for any shared services in its June 2013 submission. Nonetheless, DOD included a discussion of the first four shared services it plans to implement in fiscal year 2014, which were medical logistics, facilities planning, health information technology, and the health care plan. The information in DOD's June 2013 submission generally reflected key characteristics of business-case analyses; however, DOD did not present sufficient information to explain the basis for its cost-savings estimates. According to GAO's *Business Process Reengineering Assessment Guide*, an initial business case is essentially a high-level document aimed at convincing customers and stakeholders that reengineering the selected business process is the appropriate means for achieving performance and cost-savings goals. As the reengineering process matures, it should include detailed qualitative and quantitative analysis in support of selecting and implementing the new process that includes a statement regarding benefits, costs, and risks. DOD officials stated that the business case analyses they developed regarding the shared services to be implemented were informed by information from our previous reports on their medical governance efforts and specifically our *Business Process Reengineering Assessment Guide*.

While DOD was not required to present its business-case analyses for its shared services until its September 2013 submission, we found that the information on the four shared services included in the June 2013 submission contained a number of elements that help make the case for shared services. Specifically, the information presented included discussion of the consolidation efforts' purpose, the scope of services to be consolidated, the responsibilities of the new shared service entities, estimated implementation costs and cost savings, a timeline of events, and measures of success. DOD's submission also provided a breakdown of estimated implementation costs, with specific estimates for information technology, contractor support, personnel severance, personnel relocation, and military construction.

However, DOD's submission did not include similarly detailed quantitative analysis regarding the sources of its cost-savings estimates or provide a basis for or an explanation of key assumptions and rationales used in estimating such savings. For example, while the proposed medical logistics shared service is composed of three business lines—supplies, equipment, and housekeeping services—DOD's savings estimate is not similarly differentiated, and is presented as a single net savings range of between $132 million and $353 million from fiscal year 2014 through fiscal year 2019. Similarly, DOD's June 2013 submission states that it plans to achieve savings in administration of the TRICARE Health Plan by closing walk-in help centers and transitioning to a phone-based system and better coordinating TRICARE benefit payments with other health insurers. However, DOD's savings estimate is not similarly differentiated, and instead is presented as an aggregated net savings range of between $503 million and $787 million. As DOD moves forward with the implementation of shared services, transparent and clear business-case analyses could assist DOD in making the case for consolidation of business lines. By not providing a detailed quantitative analysis regarding the sources of cost savings in its June 2013 submission, DOD's aggregated estimate obscures the relative size, cost, and potential uncertainties or risks associated with forming a shared service. Further, the absence of such information in this submission does not allow necessary oversight of DOD's effort to benefit from a thorough understanding of how savings estimates were calculated and are planned to be achieved.

DOD also presented a risk-adjusted estimate of net cost savings for shared services based on uncertainty regarding the effectiveness of its consolidation efforts, but did not similarly consider the effect of potential increases in implementation costs. DOD's submission provides a high-level cost-savings estimate, an itemized implementation cost estimate, and a range of net savings for each of the four shared services to be implemented in fiscal year 2014. The cost-savings estimates are adjusted for risk related to the likelihood of achieving the cost savings and are presented as a range, with a 10 percent to 100 percent chance of achieving the maximum estimated savings for each shared service. Implementation costs are then subtracted from the maximum and minimum cost savings to present a range of possible net savings. According to DOD's estimates, each shared service is expected to achieve savings even when adjusted according to these risk factors. However, while DOD assessed the risk of its reforms failing to achieve their maximum potential cost savings, it did not similarly assess the risk that estimated implementation costs may increase.

DOD's past experience in managing the implementation of large scale projects demonstrates that rising implementation costs can reduce or negate potential savings. For example, as we have previously reported, after obligating approximately $2 billion over the 13-year life of its initiative to acquire an electronic health record system, as of September 2010, DOD had delivered various capabilities for outpatient care and dental care documentation, but scaled back other capabilities it had originally planned to deliver, such as replacement of legacy systems and inpatient care management. In addition, users continued to experience significant problems with the performance (speed, usability, and availability) of the portions of the system that have been deployed.[25] According to DOD's estimates, collectively, the four shared services to be implemented as part of the MHS reform in fiscal year 2014 require an investment in information-technology capabilities of about $233 million between fiscal years 2014 and 2019. According to GAO's *Business Process Reengineering Assessment Guide*, business-case analyses should demonstrate the sensitivity of the outcome to changes in assumptions, with a focus on the dominant benefit and cost elements and the areas of greatest uncertainty.[26] Given DOD's past experience in this area, rising implementation costs are an area of specific concern. Should information-technology costs or any of the other five cost categories DOD included in its estimate increase significantly, implementation costs could reduce or even negate potential cost savings.

DOD Currently Cannot Estimate How the DHA Will Affect MHS Headquarters Staff Levels

DOD's June 2013 submission was required to include the personnel levels required for the DHA and the National Capital Region (NCR) Directorate. DOD met the statutory requirement by providing a table that gave a number of personnel expected for both the DHA and specifically for the subordinate NCR Directorate. DOD's preliminary estimate of the DHA staffing as of October 1, 2013, would be 1,081 people with 42 of them specifically located within the NCR Directorate. However, DOD does not currently have the necessary information to determine how the creation of the DHA will affect the total number of MHS headquarters staff.[27] In recent years, DOD has placed increased emphasis on efficiency within its headquarters operations. For example, in 2010, the Secretary of Defense directed a departmentwide assessment of overhead, including how the department is staffed, organized, and operated, with the goal of

---

[25]GAO, *Information Technology: Opportunities Exist to Improve Management of DOD's Electronic Health Record Initiative*, GAO-11-50, (Washington, D.C.: Oct. 6, 2010).

[26]GAO/AIMD-10.1.15.

[27]According to DOD officials, MHS headquarters staff includes all personnel in commands and agencies that manage the MHS above the level of direct hospital administration.

reducing excess overhead costs and reinvesting these savings toward other priorities. The assessment identified efficiencies that were estimated to achieve about $178 billion in projected savings across the military departments and other DOD components from fiscal year 2012 through fiscal year 2016. In 2012, DOD published defense strategic guidance to direct defense priorities and spending over the coming decade stating that DOD must continue to reduce the cost of doing business, which includes finding further efficiencies in overhead and headquarters, in its business practices, and in other support activities.[28] In addition, in July 2013, the Deputy Secretary of Defense announced a 20 percent reduction in DOD management headquarters spending over 5 fiscal years beginning in fiscal year 2014. Our previous work[29] has highlighted the need for agencies to have valid, reliable data and be aware of the size of their workforce, its deployment across the organization, and the knowledge, skills, and abilities needed for the agency to pursue its mission.[30] This requirement extends beyond awareness of military and civilian personnel and includes DOD's large contractor workforce. DOD policy requires the consideration of all available personnel sources when determining manpower mix to accomplish a mission, including military and civilian personnel, as well as contractors.[31] Given the lack of current information, it is unclear what effect the DHA will have on total MHS headquarters staff levels.

When choosing among different governance models for the MHS in 2011, DOD estimated that its preferred option, which ultimately became the DHA, would save DOD $46.5 million per year in reduced personnel costs. However, while DOD officials told us in July 2013 that there will be no net increase in personnel numbers across the MHS headquarters as a result of the creation of the DHA, they do not have a numerical estimate of staffing at full operating capability. DOD's June 2013 submission includes an estimate of staffing, as required by statute, but the estimate is at the new agency's initial operating capability on October 1, 2013. According to

---

[28]Department of Defense, *Sustaining U.S. Global Leadership: Priorities for 21st Century Defense*, (Jan. 3, 2012).

[29]GAO/AIMD-10.1.15.

[30]GAO, *A Model of Strategic Human Capital Management*, GAO-02-373SP, (Washington, D.C.: March 2002).

[31]DOD Directive 1100.4, *Guidance for Manpower Management* (Feb. 12, 2005).

DOD officials, DOD's initial operating capability staff estimate includes current TRICARE Management Activity headquarters' staff, the NCR Directorate, and initial estimates of personnel for the four shared services functions DOD plans to implement in fiscal year 2014. It does not include an estimate of additional personnel for the other six shared services DOD plans to implement at a later point or any other staff necessary to reach full operating capability. Additionally, this estimate does not include any contractor positions currently associated with TRICARE Management Activity, the shared services, or other headquarters functions. Contractors form an integral part of DOD's workforce, and as noted above, DOD policy requires consideration of all sectors of the workforce when determining workforce mix, including contractors. Further, according to DOD officials, for some of these functions the number of military, civilian, and contractor staff at full operating capability could be significantly higher than the estimate of initial operating capability provided in the June 2013 submission. For example, according to a senior official responsible for information technology within the MHS, the number of staff for information technology at initial operating capability is estimated at about 400 military and civilian positions; however, that estimate increases to about 3,500 military and civilian positions and about 5,000 contractor equivalent positions at full operating capability. As a result, the submissions do not account for about 3,100 positions that may be assigned to the DHA at full operating capability.

DOD is also currently unable to estimate whether the creation of the DHA will result in an increase or decrease in DOD health care personnel because it has not completed an updated baseline assessment of MHS headquarters staff levels. DOD did conduct such a baseline assessment of its MHS headquarters staff in 2011 in order to develop cost-savings estimates as part of its examination of different possible governance models for the MHS. DOD based its decision to establish the DHA, in part, on a resulting estimate of $46.5 million in annual personnel savings, as noted above. However, according to DOD officials, the military services objected to the use of this previous baseline assessment because they believed it did not accurately reflect the current number of personnel staffed with the MHS headquarters. DOD has encountered similar issues in previous efforts to eliminate redundancies and integrate services in the MHS, such as the establishment of the Joint Task Force National Capital Region Medical (JTF CAPMED), in which officials encountered significant challenges developing an accurate, complete, and realistic joint manning document that listed all military and civilian medical personnel on board. In addition, it is unclear whether DOD plans to increase or decrease spending and reliance upon contracted full-time equivalents. DOD officials stated that while some efficiency may be achieved in headquarters staffing levels, they believe the greatest savings are to be achieved through shared services, standardization, and a more-integrated approach to the MHS as reflected in their plans for the DHA. However, by not fully describing estimated staffing levels required for implementing the reform of the governance of the MHS, DOD cannot provide decision makers with a transparent and complete picture of the military, civilian, and contractor resources that will be needed to implement the transformation. DOD officials told us that they plan to conduct a baseline assessment of headquarters staffing levels and submit a revised estimated staffing-level chart in their next required report to Congress, which was due on September 30, 2013.

Conclusions

After decades of incremental alterations to its governance structure, DOD has moved forward with an approach that it believes will increase integration and realize cost savings throughout the MHS, including an organized process for the standup of the DHA. In this context, although DOD mostly met its statutory reporting requirements in its March 2013 and June 2013 submissions, the submissions are missing key details that are important for oversight of DOD's implementation of the governance reform. Without comprehensive timelines that include interim milestones for implementation, as well as clear performance measures that are strongly linked to measurable goals and objectives, have targets, and include baseline assessments, it will be difficult for decision makers to gauge progress and identify areas requiring corrective actions. Similarly, without thoroughly explaining the sources of estimated cost savings from the implementation of its shared services projects and a means to assess the potential for cost increases, decision makers will lack visibility over the actual cost implications of implementing these projects, which could hinder their ability to achieve cost savings or adjust plans when appropriate. Finally, without a baseline assessment of current personnel numbers in MHS headquarters and an estimate of the personnel needed for DHA at full operational capability, DOD cannot provide decision makers the full scope of information they need to understand the full magnitude of implementation costs and efficiencies estimated to be gained by the reform. Until DOD provides greater clarity and transparency with regard to the performance measures, the sources of cost savings, the sensitivity of cost savings to rising implementation costs, and total staffing requirements, decision makers within DOD and Congress will not have critical information to monitor the implementation of the MHS reform effort.

Recommendations for Executive Action

To provide decision makers with more-complete information on the planned implementation, management, and oversight of DOD's newly created DHA, we recommend that the Secretary of Defense direct the Assistant Secretary of Defense (Health Affairs) to take the following five actions:

- Develop and present to Congress performance measures that are clear, quantifiable, objective, and include a baseline assessment of current performance.

- Develop and present to Congress a comprehensive timeline that includes interim milestones for all reform goals that could be used to show implementation progress.

- Provide Congress with a more-thorough explanation of the potential sources of cost savings from the implementation of its shared services projects

- Monitor implementation costs to assess whether the shared-services projects are on track to achieve projected net cost savings or if corrective actions are needed.

- Develop and present to Congress a baseline assessment of the current number of military, civilian, and contractor personnel currently working within the MHS headquarters and an estimate for DHA at full operating capability, including estimates of changes in contractor full-time equivalents.

Agency Comments

In written comments on a draft of this report, DOD concurred with our five recommendations to guide implementation of the Defense Health Agency. DOD's comments are reprinted in appendix I.

We are sending copies of this report to interested congressional committees, the Secretary of Defense, the Deputy Secretary of Defense, the Under Secretary of Defense for Personnel and Readiness, the Assistant Secretary of Defense (Health Affairs), the Defense Health Agency Director, the Surgeon General of the Air Force, the Surgeon General of the Army, and the Surgeon General of the Navy. In addition, the report is available at no charge on the GAO website at http://www.gao.gov.

If you or your staff have any questions regarding this report, please contact me at (202) 512-3604 or farrellb@gao.gov. Contact points for our Offices of Congressional Relations and Public Affairs may be found on the last page of this report. GAO staff who made key contributions to this report are listed in appendix II.

Brenda S. Farrell
Director
Defense Capabilities and Management

List of Committees

The Honorable Carl Levin
Chairman
The Honorable James N. Inhofe
Ranking Member
Committee on Armed Services
United States Senate

The Honorable Dick Durbin
Chairman
The Honorable Thad Cochran
Ranking Member
Subcommittee on Defense
Committee on Appropriations
United States Senate

The Honorable Howard P. "Buck" McKeon
Chairman
The Honorable Adam Smith
Ranking Member
Committee on Armed Services
House of Representatives

The Honorable Chairman
The Honorable Peter Visclosky
Ranking Member
Subcommittee on Defense
Committee on Appropriations
House of Representatives

Appendix I: Comments from the Department of Defense

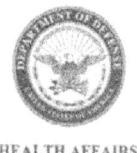

THE ASSISTANT SECRETARY OF DEFENSE

1200 DEFENSE PENTAGON
WASHINGTON, DC 20301-1200

HEALTH AFFAIRS

31 Oct 2013

Ms. Benda S. Farrell
Director, Defense Capabilities and Management
U.S. Government Accountability Office
441 G Street, N.W.
Washington, DC 20548

Dear Ms. Farrell:

This is the Department of Defense's (DoD) response to the Government Accountability Office (GAO) Draft Report, GAO-14-49 entitled DEFENSE HEALTH CARE REFORM: Additional Implementation Details Would Increase Transparency of DoD's Plans and Enhance Accountability," dated September 25, 2013 (GAO Code 351809).

Thank you for the opportunity to review and comment on the draft report. I concur with the Draft Report's findings, recommendations, and conclusion, with the following points of context: 1) the third report to Congressional Defense Committees required by section 731 of the National Defense Authorization Act for Fiscal Year (FY) 2013 addresses many of these points; and 2) with respect to the ongoing transition process from initial operating capability to full operating capability during FY 2014 and 2015, DoD expects to have opportunities to update the Congressional Defense Committees on the broad range of implementation details and progress.

My points of contact on this matter are Dr. Michel Dinneen (Functional) and Mr. Gunther Zimmerman (Audit Liaison). Dr. Dinneen may be reached at (704) 681-1724, or michael.dinneen@ha.osd.mil. Mr. Zimmerman may be reached at (703) 681-4360, or gunther.zimmerman@dha.osd.mil

Jonathan Woodson, M.D.

Appendix II: GAO Contact and Staff Acknowledgments

GAO Contact	Brenda S. Farrell, (202) 512-3604 or farrellb@gao.gov
Staff Acknowledgments	In addition to the contact named above, Lori Atkinson, Assistant Director; Rebecca Beale; Grace Coleman; Jeffrey Heit; Terry Richardson; Adam Smith; and Michael Willems made key contributions to this report.

Related GAO Products

Defense Health Care: Additional Analysis of Costs and Benefits of Potential Governance Structures is Needed, GAO-12-911 (Washington, D.C.: September 26, 2012).

Defense Health Care: Applying Key Management Practices Should Help Achieve Efficiencies within the Military Health System, GAO-12-224 (Washington, D.C.: April 12, 2012).

2012 Annual Report: Opportunities to Reduce Duplication, Overlap and Fragmentation, Achieve Savings, and Enhance Revenue, GAO-12-342SP (Washington, D.C.: Feb. 28, 2012).

Follow-up on 2011 Report, Status of Actions Taken to Reduce Duplication, Overlap, and Fragmentation, Save Tax Dollars, and Enhance Revenue, GAO-12-453SP (Washington, D.C.: Feb. 28, 2012).

Opportunities to Reduce Potential Duplication in Government Programs, Save Tax Dollars, and Enhance Revenue, GAO-11-318SP (Washington, D.C.: Mar. 1, 2011).

Military Personnel: Enhanced Collaboration and Process Improvements Needed for Determining Military Treatment Facility Medical Personnel Requirements, GAO-10-696 (Washington, D.C.: July 29, 2010).

Defense Health Care: DOD Needs to Address the Expected Benefits, Costs, and Risks for Its Newly Approved Medical Command Structure, GAO-08-122 (Washington, D.C.: Oct. 12, 2007).

Please Print on Recycled Paper.